ADMINISTRATION OF FIRST AID

Preparing for an

emergency

Dr. Juana Schumm

This book is intended to provide general information on the administration of first aid and is not a substitute for professional medical advice, diagnosis, or treatment. The author and publisher disclaim any liability, loss, or risk incurred as a consequence, directly or indirectly, of the use and application of any of the contents of this book.

Table of Content

6 | Administration of first aid

Introduction

Jenny was out hiking with her friends in a remote area when she suddenly began to experience severe chest pain and difficulty breathing. Her friends were panicked and didn't know what to do, but luckily, one of them had recently taken a first aid course and knew how to recognize the signs of a heart attack.

Thanks to her training, Jenny's friend was able to quickly call for help and provide first aid until the paramedics arrived. Because they were in a remote area, it took some time for the ambulance to reach them, but thanks to the first aid administered by her friend, Jenny was able to stay conscious and stable until help arrived. The paramedics later confirmed that she had indeed suffered a heart attack and that her friend's quick thinking and knowledge of first aid had saved her life.

This story shows how important it is to know how to administer first aid in emergency situations. You never know when you or someone you love might need it, and having the knowledge and confidence to act quickly and effectively can make all the difference in saving a life. "Administration of First Aid: Preparing for an emergency" is the perfect guide for anyone who wants to Preparing for an emergency and have the skills to make a positive difference in the world.

Administration of First Aid: Preparing for an emergency" is a comprehensive guide that teaches readers how to save lives with effective first aid administration. In today's world, it's essential to be able to act quickly in emergency situations, and knowing how to administer first aid can make all the difference in saving someone's life.

This book provides an in-depth overview of the basic principles of first aid, common emergencies, advanced first aid techniques, first aid kits and equipment, and special situations and considerations.

Chapter 1 explores the basic principles of first aid, including understanding the ABCs of first aid, when to call for help, and personal safety measures. This chapter sets the foundation for the rest of the book, ensuring that readers understand the importance of acting quickly and safely in emergency situations.

Chapter 2 delves into the most common emergencies and their management. It covers how to care for wounds, bleeding, burns, choking, fractures, sprains, heat exhaustion, and hypothermia, among others. This chapter also provides readers with information on how to recognize the signs and symptoms of these emergencies and how to respond effectively.

Chapter 3 focuses on advanced first aid techniques, such as CPR, the use of Automated External Defibrillators (AEDs), head and spinal injuries, seizures and convulsions, and allergic reactions and anaphylaxis. This chapter provides detailed step-by-step instructions on how to perform each technique, making it easy for readers to learn and practice.

Chapter 4 covers first aid kits and equipment, including the essential items to include in a first aid kit, how to maintain and restock a kit, and how to store and transport it safely.

Chapter 5 explores special situations and considerations, such as administering first aid to children and infants, the elderly, and in natural disasters and emergencies. This chapter also covers psychological first aid and how to care for someone who has experienced trauma.

This book recaps the key points covered in each chapter and encourages readers to learn and practice first aid skills. The appendices provide emergency contact information, a glossary of terms, and additional resources and references for further learning.

Overall, "Administration of First Aid: Preparing for an emergency" is an essential guide for anyone who wants to learn how to administer first aid effectively. Whether you are a medical professional, a parent, or just someone who wants to be prepared for emergencies, this book will give you the knowledge and confidence to act quickly and save lives.

If you want to Preparing for an emergency and have the knowledge and skills to save lives in emergency situations, "Administration of First Aid: Preparing for an emergency" is the book for you! With its comprehensive coverage of basic and advanced first aid techniques, common emergencies, first aid kits and equipment, and special situations and considerations, this book provides you with the tools you need to act quickly and confidently in any emergency.

Don't wait until it's too late to learn how to administer first aid effectively. Take action now and get your copy of "Administration of First Aid: Preparing for an emergency". With its clear, step-by-step instructions, practical advice, and real-world examples, this book will empower you to be a lifesaver and make a positive difference in the world. Order your copy today and Preparing for an emergency

"The Administration of First Aid: Preparing for an emergency" is an essential guide for anyone looking to learn how to respond to emergencies and provide initial medical care.

The book covers a wide range of topics, including assessing the situation, identifying the injury or illness, and providing the appropriate first aid treatment.

The author's comprehensive approach to first aid is evident throughout the book. The step-by-step instructions and illustrations make it easy for readers to understand and apply the techniques in real-life situations. Additionally, the author emphasizes the importance of being prepared for emergencies by providing information on first aid kits, emergency plans, and basic safety tips.

What sets this book apart from other first aid guides is its focus on both physical and psychological first aid. The author recognizes that emergencies can be traumatic and stressful, and includes guidance on how to provide emotional support to those in need.

Overall, "The Administration of First Aid: Preparing for an emergency" is a valuable resource for anyone looking to be better prepared for emergencies. It provides the knowledge and skills needed to respond confidently and effectively in a crisis, potentially saving lives and minimizing the impact of injuries and illnesses. I highly recommend this book to anyone interested in learning first aid or looking to refresh their existing skills.

In conclusion, knowing first aid is essential because accidents can happen at any time and any place. Being trained in first aid can mean the difference between life and death in some situations. It is important to be prepared and have the knowledge and skills needed to provide basic medical care until professional help arrives.

The Importance of Acting Quickly

In an emergency situation, every second counts. The ability to act quickly and efficiently can often mean the difference between life and death. This is especially true when it comes to administering first aid.

First aid is the initial assistance given to someone who is injured or suddenly becomes ill before professional medical help arrives. It can be as simple as applying a bandage to a small wound or as complex as administering CPR to someone who has stopped breathing.

The importance of acting quickly in administering first aid cannot be overstated. The first few minutes after an injury or illness can be critical, and the right intervention can make all the difference.

For example, in the case of a severe bleeding injury, every minute counts in controlling the bleeding. Applying direct pressure to the wound and elevating the affected limb can help slow down the bleeding and give the injured person a better chance of survival.

Similarly, if someone is experiencing chest pains or difficulty breathing, administering first aid quickly can be the difference between life and death. The sooner the person receives proper medical care, the better the chances of survival and recovery.

Additionally, quick administration of first aid can also prevent further injury or complications. For example, in the case of a fractured bone, immobilizing the affected limb with a splint or brace can prevent further damage to the surrounding tissues and help reduce pain.

It's important to note that administering first aid quickly does not mean administering it haphazardly. It's crucial to follow proper protocols and procedures to ensure that the injured or ill person receives the best possible care.

In conclusion, acting quickly in administering first aid is critical in an emergency situation. Whether it's controlling bleeding, providing CPR, or immobilizing a fracture, every second counts in providing the best possible outcome. By being prepared, remaining calm, and knowing what to do in an emergency, you can help save lives and prevent further injury.

18 | Administration of first aid

Chapter 1: Basic Principles of First Aid

Understanding the ABCs of First Aid

First Aid refers to the initial assistance given to someone who has suffered an injury or illness before professional medical help arrives. It is essential to have basic knowledge of First Aid techniques to be prepared in case of an emergency. Here are some of the ABCs of First Aid:

A - Airway: Ensure that the airway of the injured person is clear, and they are able to breathe. If the person is unconscious, check for any obstruction in the mouth or throat, and clear it if possible. If the person is not breathing, start CPR (cardiopulmonary resuscitation) immediately.

B - Breathing: Check for breathing by looking, listening, and feeling for signs of chest movement, breath sounds, and air coming from the nose or mouth. If the person is not breathing, start CPR.

C - Circulation: Check for a pulse and signs of blood circulation. If the person has no pulse or is not breathing, start CPR immediately. If there is bleeding, apply pressure to the wound to control the bleeding.

D - Disability: Check for any signs of disability, such as confusion or loss of consciousness, which could indicate a head injury or other serious condition.

E - Exposure: Check for any exposure to extreme temperatures, chemicals, or other hazards, and take appropriate action to prevent further harm.

It is essential to remember that First Aid is not a substitute for professional medical care. It is only meant to provide initial assistance until medical help arrives. Therefore, it is important to call emergency services as soon as possible and follow their instructions. Additionally, it is important to take a First Aid course to learn proper techniques and procedures.

When to Call for Help

One of the most important principles in administering first aid is knowing when to call for professional medical help. This is critical because certain injuries and medical emergencies require immediate medical attention beyond what can be provided by basic first aid.

Here are some situations where you should call for medical help:

1. The person is unconscious or unresponsive.

2. The person is having difficulty breathing or has stopped breathing.

3. The person is experiencing severe chest pain or pressure.

4. The person is bleeding heavily and the bleeding does not stop with direct pressure.

5. When you notice that the person has a seizure that last more than five (5) minutes.

6. The person has ingested poison or overdosed on medication.

7. The person has a severe allergic reaction (anaphylaxis).

8. The person has a head injury and is vomiting or has lost consciousness.

9. The person has a broken bone that is visibly deformed or protruding through the skin.

In general, if you are unsure if you should call for medical help, it is always better to err on the side of caution and seek professional medical attention. Remember that prompt medical attention can often mean the difference between life and death, so don't hesitate to call for help when you need it

Personal Safety Measures

Administering first aid can be an important skill to have in emergencies, but it is important to keep yourself safe while providing aid to someone else. Here are some personal safety measures to apply when administering first aid:

1. **Assess the situation:** Before you start administering first aid, make sure that the area around you is safe. Look for any hazards, such as broken glass, sharp objects, or electrical wires, and move the injured person to a safe location if possible.

2. **Use personal protective equipment:** When providing first aid, it is important to protect yourself from exposure to blood or bodily fluids. Wear gloves, eye protection, and a mask if possible.

3. **Wash your hands:** Before and after administering first aid, make sure to wash your hands thoroughly with soap and water to prevent the spread of germs.

4. **Communicate with the injured person:** Before providing any aid, ask the injured person if they are okay with you providing assistance. Communicate with them throughout the process and ask them to inform you of any changes in their condition.

5. **Use proper technique:** When providing first aid, make sure to use proper technique to avoid injury to yourself or the injured person. For example, when performing CPR, make sure to keep your hands and arms straight and use your upper body strength to compress the chest.

6. **Do not move the injured person unnecessarily:** Unless it is necessary to move the injured person to a safe location, avoid moving them as this could cause further injury.

By following these personal safety measures, you can help ensure that you are able to provide effective first aid while keeping yourself safe.

Chapter 2: Common Emergencies and Their Management

Bleeding and Wound Care

The first step in treating bleeding and wound care is to make sure that you and the injured person are safe. If the wound is serious, it's important to call for emergency medical assistance.

Here are some general steps you can take for bleeding and wound care:

1. **Apply pressure:** Use a clean cloth or bandage to apply pressure to the wound. If the cloth becomes soaked with blood, add more layers on top.

2. **Elevate the injured area:** If possible, raise the injured area above the heart to slow down bleeding.

3. **Clean the wound:** Once bleeding has slowed or stopped, gently clean the wound with soap and water. If the wound is deep, it may require irrigation with sterile saline solution.

4. **Cover the wound:** After cleaning the wound, apply an antibiotic ointment and cover it with a sterile bandage or dressing.

5. **Monitor the wound:** Check the wound regularly for signs of infection, such as redness, swelling, or discharge.

6. **Seek medical attention:** If the bleeding is severe, the wound is deep, or you suspect an infection, seek medical attention right away.

It's important to note that different wounds may require different treatments, and it's always best to follow the advice of a medical professional. Additionally, if someone is bleeding profusely or has a wound that won't stop bleeding, call for emergency medical assistance immediately.

Burns and Scalds

When providing first aid for burns and scalds, the first priority is to remove the person from the source of the burn, such as a hot surface or boiling liquid. Here are the general steps for treating a burn or scald:

1. **Cool the burn:** Run cool water over the burn for at least 10-20 minutes, or until the pain subsides. Do not use ice or very cold water, as this can damage the skin further.

2. **Remove any clothing or jewelry from the affected area:** unless it is sticking to the skin.

3. **If it is sticking to the skin:** leave it in place to avoid further damage.

4. **Cover the burn:** Cover the burn with a clean, sterile dressing or a clean, non-fluffy material such as plastic wrap or a clean plastic bag.

5. **Take pain relief medication:** Over-the-counter pain relief medication such as acetaminophen or ibuprofen can help to relieve pain and reduce inflammation.

6. **Seek medical attention:** Seek medical attention for large or deep burns, burns that affect the face, hands, feet or genitals, or if the person shows signs of shock, such as

pale or clammy skin, rapid breathing, or a rapid heartbeat.

It's important to note that if the burn is severe or covers a large area of the body, do not try to cool it with water or remove any clothing that is stuck to the skin. In these cases, seek medical attention immediately.

Choking and Suffocation

Choking and suffocation are emergency situations that require immediate action. Here are the general steps for treating choking and suffocation:

1. **Call for emergency medical assistance:** If the person is choking or suffocating, call for emergency medical assistance right away.

2. **Perform the Heimlich maneuver:** If the person is conscious and choking, stand behind them and wrap your arms around

their waist. Make a fist with one hand and place it just above the person's belly button. Grasp the fist with your other hand and give quick upward thrusts until the object is dislodged.

3. **Clear the airway**: If the person is unconscious, check their mouth for any visible obstructions and clear them if possible. If you can't see the object, perform CPR until medical help arrives.

4. **Perform rescue breathing:** If the person is not breathing, tilt their head back and lift their chin to open their airway. Pinch their nose and give two breaths, watching for the chest to rise.

5. **Monitor the person's condition:** Continue to monitor the person's breathing and pulse until emergency medical help arrives.

It's important to note that if the person is unconscious, do not try to clear the airway with your fingers as this can push the object further down the throat. Instead, perform rescue breathing until medical help arrives.

Additionally, it's important to take steps to prevent choking and suffocation, such as cutting food into small pieces and supervising young children and infants at all times.

Fractures and Sprains

Fractures and sprains are injuries that can be very painful and require immediate attention. Here are the general steps for treating fractures and sprains:

1. **Stop any bleeding:** If there is any bleeding, apply pressure to the wound with a clean cloth or bandage.

2. **Immobilize the injured area:** Use a splint or brace to immobilize the injured area and prevent further damage. If you don't have a splint or brace, use a rolled-up newspaper or magazine.

3. **Apply ice:** Apply an ice pack or a cold compress to the injured area to help reduce swelling and pain.

4. **Elevate the injured area:** If possible, elevate the injured area above the heart to reduce swelling.

5. **Take pain relief medication:** Over-the-counter pain relief medication such as acetaminophen or ibuprofen can help to relieve pain and reduce inflammation.

6. **Seek medical attention:** Seek medical attention for any suspected fractures, as they may require X-rays and further treatment.

It's important to note that if the person has a suspected spinal injury, do not attempt to move them unless it is absolutely necessary to prevent further injury or to administer CPR. Additionally, if the person has a suspected head injury or loss of consciousness, seek medical attention immediately.

Heat Exhaustion and Heatstroke

Heat exhaustion and heatstroke are serious conditions that can occur when a person is exposed to high temperatures for an extended period of time. Here are the general steps for treating heat exhaustion and heatstroke:

1. **Move the person to a cooler location:** Move the person to a cooler location, preferably indoors with air conditioning or

in the shade. Remove any excess clothing and loosen tight clothing.

2. **Hydrate the person:** Have the person drink cool, non-alcoholic beverages such as water or sports drinks that contain electrolytes.

3. **Cool the person down:** Apply cool water to the person's skin with a damp cloth or spray bottle, or use a fan to increase air circulation. If possible, immerse the person in a cool bath or shower.

4. **Monitor the person's condition:** Stay with the person and monitor his/her condition. Watch for signs of worsening symptoms, such as confusion or seizures.

5. **Seek medical attention:** Seek medical attention immediately if the person's condition does not improve, or if they show

signs of heatstroke such as a body temperature of 103°F (39.4°C) or higher, rapid heartbeat, rapid breathing, confusion, or loss of consciousness.

It's important to note that prevention is key when it comes to heat exhaustion and heatstroke. Stay hydrated, avoid prolonged exposure to high temperatures, wear lightweight and loose-fitting clothing, and take frequent breaks in the shade or indoors with air conditioning.

Hypothermia and Frostbite

Hypothermia and frostbite are both conditions that can occur when a person is exposed to cold temperatures for an extended period of time.

For hypothermia, the first aid treatment includes:

1. Move the person to a warm and dry location immediately.

2. Remove any wet cloth and replace with a dry cloth or blanket.

3. Cover the person's head and neck with a hat or scarf.

4. Wrap the person in warm blankets or a sleeping bag to help raise the body temperature.

5. If the person is conscious, give them warm liquids like soup, tea, or warm water (avoid alcohol and caffeine).

6. If the person is unconscious or not breathing, seek emergency medical attention and perform CPR if necessary.

For frostbite, the first aid treatment includes:

1. Move the person to a warm and dry location immediately.

2. Remove any wet cloth and replace with a dry cloth or blanket.

3. Immerse the affected area in warm (not hot) water for 15-30 minutes, or until the skin color returns to normal.

4. Do not rub the affected area or apply direct heat, such as a heating pad or hot water bottle.

5. Elevate the affected area to reduce swelling.

6. If the person is experiencing severe frostbite or hypothermia symptoms, seek emergency medical attention immediately.

It's important to note that both hypothermia and frostbite are serious conditions that require prompt medical attention. If you suspect someone is experiencing these conditions, call for emergency medical services right away.

Chapter 3: Advanced First Aid Techniques

Cardio-Pulmonary Resuscitation (CPR)

Cardio-Pulmonary Resuscitation (CPR) is a first aid technique used to revive a person who has stopped breathing or whose heart has stopped beating. CPR involves a combination of chest compressions and rescue breaths to keep blood flowing and oxygen circulating in the body until medical help arrives.

Here's how to perform CPR:

1. **Check for responsiveness:** First, check to see if the person is responding. Tap their shoulders and shout their name. If there is

no response, then the person is unconscious and you need to perform CPR.

2. **Call for help:** Call emergency services immediately or ask someone nearby to call for you. The sooner you can get professional help, the better the chances of survival.

3. **Position the person:** Carefully roll the person onto their back and make sure their airway is open. To do this, tilt their head back slightly and lift their chin. This will help to clear any obstructions and make it easier for air to pass through.

4. **Begin chest compressions:** Place the heel of your hand on the center of the person's chest (between the nipples) and interlock your fingers. Press down firmly and quickly, compressing the chest by about 2 inches.

Perform 30 compressions at a rate of about 100-120 compressions per minute.

5. **Provide rescue breaths:** After the chest compressions, tilt the person's head back and lift their chin.

Pinch their nose closed and breathe into their mouth for about one second to provide rescue breaths. You should see their chest rise as you do this. Repeat this step twice.

Continue cycles of chest compressions and rescue breaths: Repeat the cycle of 30 chest compressions followed by two rescue breaths until professional help arrives or the person starts to show signs of recovery.

Remember, performing CPR can be tiring, so it's important to switch with someone else if possible. Also, keep in mind that CPR should only be performed by trained individuals who have been certified in CPR. If you are not certified, provide basic first aid until medical help arrives.

Use of Automated External Defibrillators (AEDs)

Automated External Defibrillators (AEDs) are portable electronic devices used to treat sudden cardiac arrest (SCA) by delivering an electric shock to the heart in order to restore its normal rhythm. AEDs are designed to be easy to use by non-medical personnel, and can greatly increase the chances of survival for a person experiencing SCA.

When using an AED, it is important to follow the following advance first aid techniques:

1. **Call for Emergency Medical Services (EMS) immediately:** If someone is found unconscious or unresponsive, the first step is to call for emergency medical services.

Time is of the essence when dealing with SCA, and quick action can greatly increase the chances of survival.

2. **Begin CPR:** If the person is not breathing or has no pulse, begin CPR (Cardiopulmonary Resuscitation) immediately. This involves giving chest compressions and rescue breaths to circulate oxygenated blood to the brain and other organs until the AED arrives.

3. **Turn on the AED:** Once the AED arrives, turn it on and follow the voice prompts. The device will guide you through the steps to attach the electrode pads to the person's chest.

4. **Clear the area:** Before delivering a shock, make sure that everyone is clear of the person's body to avoid injury.

5. **Deliver the shock:** Once the electrode pads are in place, the AED will analyze the person's heart rhythm and determine if a shock is necessary.

6. **If it is a shock:** make sure that no one is touching the person and press the shock button as directed by the device.

7. **Resume CPR:** After delivering a shock, resume CPR immediately for two minutes before the AED reanalyzes the person's heart rhythm and determines if another shock is needed.

It is important to note that AEDs are safe and effective when used properly, and can greatly increase the chances of survival for a person experiencing SCA. However, they are only one part of the chain of survival, and prompt activation of

EMS, early CPR, and rapid defibrillation are all critical components of successful resuscitation.

Head and Spinal Injuries

Head and spinal injuries are serious medical emergencies that require immediate attention.

In many cases, these types of injuries can be life-threatening or lead to permanent disability if not treated properly. Therefore, it is important to follow advanced first aid techniques when treating head and spinal injuries.

1. **Call for Emergency Medical Services (EMS) immediately:** If someone has sustained a head or spinal injury, it is essential to call for EMS immediately. The patient will require medical attention and transportation to a hospital.

2. **Ensure Airway, Breathing, and Circulation (ABC):** Check the person's airway, breathing, and circulation. Ensure that the airway is open, and the person is breathing. If the person is not breathing, initiate CPR (Cardiopulmonary Resuscitation).

3. **Stabilize the Neck:** If there is a suspected spinal injury, the person's neck must be stabilized to prevent further damage.

4. **Do not move the person's head or neck:** This can cause additional spinal injury. Hold the person's head and neck in place and use a cervical collar if available.

5. **Assess the Injury:** Assess the extent of the injury and look for any signs of a head or spinal injury, such as swelling, bleeding, or deformity.

6. **Control Bleeding:** If there is any bleeding, apply pressure to the wound to control the bleeding. Do not move the person's head or neck while doing this.

7. **Maintain Body Temperature:** If the person is exposed to cold or hot temperatures, cover the person with a blanket or coat to maintain body temperature.

8. **Monitor Vital Signs:** Monitor the person's vital signs, including breathing rate, pulse, and blood pressure. Be prepared to administer first aid for any changes in vital signs, such as shock or cardiac arrest.

9. **Keep the Person Calm and Comfortable:** Reassure the person and keep them calm and comfortable. Do not administer any medications or fluids unless directed to do so by a medical professional.

It is important to note that head and spinal injuries are serious and should be treated by trained medical professionals as soon as possible. While waiting for EMS to arrive, following these advanced first aid techniques can help prevent further injury and potentially save the person's life

Seizures and Convulsions

Seizures and convulsions can be a frightening experience both for the person having the seizure and for any bystanders who witness it. If you ever find yourself in a situation where someone is having a seizure, here are the steps you can take to provide advanced first aid:

1. Stay calm and assess the situation. Most seizures are brief and do not require medical attention, but it's important to monitor the person's condition to ensure that they are

breathing properly and not injuring themselves during the seizure.

2. Protect the person from injury. Move any nearby objects that could cause harm, such as furniture or sharp objects.

3. If the person is convulsing, gently turn them onto their side to prevent choking or aspiration of saliva or vomit. Do not restrain or hold them down during the seizure.

4. Call for medical assistance if the seizure lasts longer than 5 minutes or if it is the person's first seizure. Call an ambulance if the person is injured or if they are pregnant, have diabetes, or have a history of heart disease.

5. After the seizure ends, keep the person on their side and monitor their breathing and

pulse. Do not give them anything to eat or drink until they are fully alert and able to swallow safely.

6. If the person is unconscious or not breathing after the seizure, begin CPR immediately.

7. It is advisable you with the person until adequate medical help arrives.

In summary, the key to providing advanced first aid for seizures and convulsions is to remain calm, protect the person from injury, and call for medical assistance if needed. With prompt and appropriate care, most people recover fully from seizures and convulsions without complications.

Allergic Reactions and Anaphylaxis

Allergic reactions and anaphylaxis can be life-threatening emergencies that require immediate medical attention. As a first aider, you can take the following steps to help someone who is experiencing an allergic reaction or anaphylaxis:

1. **Recognize the symptoms:** Symptoms of an allergic reaction can include hives, swelling of the face, lips, tongue or throat, difficulty breathing, wheezing, rapid heartbeat, and a feeling of impending doom. In some severe cases, the person may become unconscious.

2. **Call for emergency medical assistance:** Call for an ambulance or activate the emergency response system in your area. Anaphylaxis is a medical emergency that requires an immediate treatment.

3. **Administer an epinephrine auto-injector (EAI):** If the person has an EAI prescribed by their doctor, help them to use it immediately. Epinephrine is a medication that can help to reverse the symptoms of an

allergic reaction by constricting blood vessels and relaxing airway muscles.

4. **Help the person to lie down:** If the person is feeling faint or has difficulty breathing, help them to lie down with their legs elevated. This can improve blood flow to the brain and ease breathing.

5. **Monitor the person's vital signs:** Keep an eye on the person's breathing, pulse, and level of consciousness. Be prepared to start CPR if the person stops breathing or their heart stops beating.

6. **Provide reassurance and support**: Remain calm and reassure the person that help is on the way. Encourage them to stay calm and relaxed as this can help to reduce the severity of the allergic reaction.

7. **Avoid giving the person anything to eat or drink:** Do not offer the person anything to eat or drink as this can worsen the symptoms of an allergic reaction.

8. **Stay with the person until medical help arrives:** Stay with the person until emergency medical services arrive. Be prepared to provide additional first aid as needed.

Remember that early recognition and prompt treatment of an allergic reaction or anaphylaxis can be life-saving. If you suspect that someone is having an allergic reaction or anaphylaxis, do not hesitate to call for emergency medical assistance.

Chapter 4: First Aid Kits and Equipment

Essential Items to Include in a First Aid Kit

A first aid kit is an essential item that every home, workplace, and vehicle should have. It contains basic medical supplies and equipment that can be used to treat minor injuries and illnesses. Here are some essential items that should be included in a first aid kit:

1. Adhesive bandages of various sizes

2. Sterile gauze pads and rolls

3. Medical tape

4. Antiseptic wipes or solution

5. Alcohol wipes

6. Disposable gloves

7. Tweezers

8. Scissors

9. Instant cold packs

10. Thermometer

11. Pain relievers such as aspirin or ibuprofen

12. Antihistamines for allergic reactions

13. Hydrocortisone cream for itching or rashes

14. Calamine lotion for skin irritation

15. Anti-diarrheal medication

16. Oral rehydration salts

17. Sterile eyewash and eye pads

18. Breathing barrier devices for CPR

19. First aid manual or instruction booklet

It's important to check the contents of your first aid kit regularly to ensure that everything is up-to-date and in good condition. Replace any expired or damaged items and add additional supplies as needed based on your individual needs and situation.

Maintaining and Restocking Your Kit

Maintaining and restocking your first aid kit is essential to ensure that it is always ready to use in the event of an emergency. Here are some steps to follow for maintaining and restocking your first aid kit:

1. **Check the expiration dates:** The first step is to check the expiration dates of all items in your first aid kit. Remove any expired items and replace them with new ones.

2. **Clean and organize the kit:** Clean the first aid kit thoroughly, and organize the items in a way that makes them easy to find. Consider using compartments or labels to keep everything in its place.

3. **Assess your needs:** Think about the types of injuries or emergencies that you are most likely to encounter and make sure your kit is equipped to handle them. For example, if you spend a lot of time outdoors, you may want to include insect repellent or sunscreen in your kit.

4. **Restock essential items:** Make sure you have an ample supply of essential items, such as bandages, gauze, adhesive tape, antiseptic wipes, and pain relievers. These are items that you will likely use frequently, so you want to make sure you always have enough on hand.

5. **Consider additional items:** Depending on your needs, you may want to consider including additional items such as a thermometer, instant cold packs, scissors, tweezers, and a flashlight.

6. **Keep it visible and accessible:** Store your first aid kit in a visible and easily accessible location. Make sure everyone in your household knows where it is and how to use it.

7. **Regularly check and update:** Check your first aid kit regularly to ensure that it remains fully stocked and up to date. This is especially important if you use items from the kit frequently.

By following these steps, you can ensure that your first aid kit is always ready to use and that you have everything you need to handle common injuries and emergencies.

Chapter 5: Special Situations and Considerations

First Aid for Children and Infants

Administering first aid to children and infants requires special considerations and precautions. Here are some of the special situations and considerations to keep in mind when providing first aid to children and infants:

1. **Age-appropriate techniques:** When providing first aid to children and infants, it is important to use age-appropriate techniques. The methods used for adults may not be suitable for children and infants due to their smaller size and developing anatomy.

2. **Emotional considerations:** Children and infants may be frightened or in pain, so it is important to provide emotional support and reassurance throughout the first aid process.

3. **Communication:** Children and infants may not be able to communicate their symptoms or needs effectively. Therefore, it is important to observe their behavior and look for signs of distress.

4. **Anatomical differences:** Children and infants have anatomical differences compared to adults. For example, their airways are smaller and more easily obstructed. Therefore, techniques such as CPR and the Heimlich maneuver must be modified for children and infants.

5. **Dosage considerations:** Dosages for medications and other treatments may vary

based on the weight and age of the child or infant.

6. **Consult a medical professional:** It is important to consult a medical professional or pediatrician before administering any medication.

7. **Allergic reactions:** Children and infants may have allergies that are not yet known. Therefore, it is important to be aware of any potential allergens and to have an emergency plan in case of an allergic reaction.

8. **Suspected abuse:** In cases where abuse or neglect is suspected, it is important to follow the appropriate reporting procedures and provide first aid with sensitivity and compassion.

9. **Caregiver involvement:** In most cases, a caregiver or parent should be present when administering first aid to a child or infant. The caregiver can provide additional information and support and help ensure that the child or infant receives appropriate medical attention.

By being aware of these special situations and considerations, you can provide effective and safe first aid to children and infants. It is always recommended to take a first aid course that includes specific training on providing first aid to children and infants.

First Aid for the Elderly

Administering first aid to the elderly requires special considerations and precautions due to age-related changes in their bodies. Here are some of the special situations and considerations to keep in mind when providing first aid to the elderly:

1. **Frailty and mobility:** Elderly individuals may be frailer or have limited mobility. When providing first aid, it is important to take care not to cause any additional harm, such as by moving the individual inappropriately or using excessive force.

2. **Medications:** Elderly individuals may be taking multiple medications, which can increase the risk of interactions or side effects. When providing first aid, it is important to be aware of any medications the individual is taking and to consult a

medical professional before administering any additional medications.

3. **Cognitive impairment:** Elderly individuals may have cognitive impairment, which can affect their ability to communicate or understand instructions. When providing first aid, it may be necessary to use alternative communication methods or seek assistance from a caregiver or medical professional.

4. **Chronic conditions:** Elderly individuals may have chronic conditions such as diabetes, heart disease, or respiratory problems that can complicate first aid treatment. It is important to be aware of any chronic conditions and to consult a medical professional if necessary.

5. **Dementia or Alzheimer's disease:** Elderly individuals with dementia or Alzheimer's disease may become confused or agitated during first aid treatment. It is important to approach these situations with patience and understanding and to seek assistance from a caregiver or medical professional as needed.

6. **Sensory impairments:** Elderly individuals may have sensory impairments, such as hearing or vision loss, which can affect their ability to communicate or understand instructions. It is important to use clear and concise communication and to be aware of any potential communication barriers.

7. **Falls:** Elderly individuals are at an increased risk of falls, which can result in injuries such as fractures or head injuries. When providing first aid for falls, it is important to

assess the individual for any injuries and to seek medical attention if necessary.

By being aware of these special situations and considerations, you can provide effective and safe first aid to the elderly. It is always recommended to take a first aid course that includes specific training on providing first aid to the elderly.

First Aid in Natural Disasters and Emergencies

Administering first aid in natural disasters and emergencies requires special considerations and precautions due to the challenging and unpredictable nature of these situations. Here are some of the special situations and considerations to keep in mind when providing first aid in natural disasters and emergencies:

1. **Safety:** The safety of the first aid provider and the victim must be the top priority in any emergency situation. The first aid provider must assess the situation and take appropriate safety measures before providing first aid.

2. **Communication:** Communication is often challenging during natural disasters and emergencies due to power outages, downed phone lines, and other factors. It is important to have alternative communication methods and to use clear and concise instructions when providing first aid.

3. **Resources:** Natural disasters and emergencies can disrupt the supply chain for medical supplies and equipment. The first aid provider must be resourceful and use whatever materials are available to provide first aid.

4. **Triage:** In mass casualty situations, it may be necessary to prioritize care based on the severity of injuries or illnesses. The first aid provider must be able to quickly assess victims and provide appropriate care.

5. **Emotional trauma:** Natural disasters and emergencies can cause emotional trauma for victims and first aid providers. It is important to provide emotional support and reassurance as well as physical first aid.

6. **Environmental factors:** Natural disasters and emergencies can expose victims and first aid providers to extreme weather conditions, hazardous materials, and other environmental factors. The first aid provider must take appropriate precautions to protect themselves and the victim.

7. **Displacement:** Natural disasters and emergencies can cause displacement of people from their homes and communities. The first aid provider must be aware of any cultural or language barriers and be sensitive to the needs of displaced individuals

By being aware of these special situations and considerations, you can provide effective and safe first aid in natural disasters and emergencies. It is always recommended to take a first aid course that includes specific training on providing first aid in emergency situations.

Psychological First Aid

Psychological first aid (PFA) is a form of first aid that focuses on providing emotional and psychological support to individuals who have experienced a traumatic event or are in a crisis situation. Here are some of the special situations and considerations to keep in mind when administering psychological first aid:

1. **Safety:** The safety of the first aid provider and the person receiving psychological first aid must be the top priority. The first aid provider must assess the situation and take appropriate safety measures before providing psychological first aid.

2. **Communication:** Clear and effective communication is crucial in psychological first aid. The first aid provider must use clear and concise language and be sensitive to any cultural or language barriers.

3. **Trauma:** Individuals who have experienced a traumatic event may be experiencing a range of emotions, including shock, fear, anger, and sadness.

The first aid provider must be able to recognize the signs of trauma and provide appropriate support.

4. **Resilience:** Psychological first aid should focus on promoting resilience and coping strategies. The first aid provider should help the individual identify their strengths and resources, and develop a plan for moving forward.

5. **Cultural sensitivity:** Cultural sensitivity is crucial in psychological first aid. The first aid provider must be aware of any cultural differences and be sensitive to the individual's cultural background and beliefs.

6. **Confidentiality:** Psychological first aid should be provided in a confidential and non-judgmental manner. The first aid provider must respect the individual's

privacy and ensure that any information shared is kept confidential.

7. **Referrals:** Psychological first aid should be a short-term intervention. The first aid provider should be able to recognize when additional support is needed and make appropriate referrals to mental health professionals.

8. **Self-care:** Providing psychological first aid can be emotionally taxing. The first aid provider must practice self-care and seek support if needed.

By being aware of these special situations and considerations, you can provide effective and safe psychological first aid. It is always recommended to take a psychological first aid course that includes specific training on providing emotional and psychological support in crisis situations.

Conclusion

Administration of First Aid: Preparing for an emergency" is a comprehensive guidebook that equips readers with the knowledge and skills needed to handle a variety of emergency situations. The book comprises five chapters, each of which covers a crucial aspect of first aid administration.

Chapter 1 provides an overview of the basic principles of first aid, including the key concepts of assessing the situation, ensuring safety, and providing initial care. The chapter also explores the importance of obtaining a detailed medical history and communicating effectively with emergency services.

Chapter 2 delves into the most common emergencies, such as cardiac arrest, bleeding, and shock, and provides practical guidance on their management. The chapter includes step-by-step instructions on how to perform CPR, control bleeding, and stabilize a patient in shock.

Chapter 3 focuses on advanced first-aid techniques that may be required in more complex emergency situations, such as spinal injuries, fractures, and head trauma. The chapter covers the use of advanced equipment, such as cervical collars, splints, and traction devices, and emphasizes the importance of effective communication and teamwork.

Chapter 4 covers first aid kits and equipment, including the types of supplies that should be included in a basic first aid kit, and how to select and maintain medical equipment for emergency situations.

Chapter 5 explores special situations and considerations, such as dealing with infants and children, responding to environmental emergencies, and providing first aid in remote or hazardous environments. The chapter also discusses the legal and ethical considerations that are relevant to administering first aid.

Overall, "Administration of First Aid: Preparing for an emergency" is an essential guide for anyone who wants to be prepared for emergencies and is seeking to gain a comprehensive understanding of first aid principles, techniques, and equipment.

80 | Administration of first aid

Recap of Key Points

Here are some key points from each chapter of the book "Administration of First Aid: Preparing for an emergency":

Chapter 1: Basic Principles of First Aid

Always prioritize personal and bystander safety when providing first aid

Assess the situation before administering any treatment

Follow the ABCs of first aid: Airway, Breathing, Circulation

Treat the most life-threatening injuries or conditions first

Seek professional medical help when needed

Chapter 2: Common Emergencies and Their Management

Learn the signs and symptoms of common emergencies, such as cardiac arrest, choking, and severe bleeding

Understand how to perform basic life support (BLS), including CPR and the use of an automated external defibrillator (AED)

Know how to treat wounds and injuries, such as burns, fractures, and sprains

Understand the basics of managing medical emergencies, such as allergic reactions, seizures, and stroke

Chapter 3: Advanced First-Aid Techniques

Learn advanced techniques for managing emergencies, such as administering medication, performing advanced airway management, and providing oxygen therapy

Understand how to manage more complex medical emergencies, such as childbirth, hypothermia, and hyperthermia

Learn how to properly use and administer first aid equipment, such as splints and bandages.

Chapter 4: First Aid Kits and Equipment

Understand what should be included in a basic first aid kit.

Know how to use each item in a first aid kit, such as bandages, antiseptics, and medications

Learn how to properly maintain and store a first aid kit

Chapter 5: Special Situations and Considerations

Understand how to provide first aid in special situations, such as during natural disasters or in remote areas

Learn how to provide first aid to specific populations, such as infants, children, and the elderly

Understand how to provide first aid to individuals with disabilities or special needs

Overall, "Administration of First Aid: Preparing for an emergency" provides a comprehensive overview of first aid principles, techniques, and equipment that can help anyone respond to emergencies with confidence and skill.

Encouragement to Learn and Practice First Aid Skills

Learning and practicing first aid skills is an incredibly valuable and important skillset for anyone to have. Accidents and emergencies can happen at any time and having the ability to provide immediate and appropriate first aid can make all the difference in saving someone's life or preventing further injury.

Encouraging people to learn and practice first aid skills is essential as it can have a profound impact on their own lives, as well as the lives of others around them. Knowing what to do in an emergency can give individuals the confidence and ability to take quick action, potentially saving someone's life or minimizing the severity of an injury.

By learning first aid skills, individuals can also become more prepared for unexpected situations. Whether it is a small injury or a more significant emergency, having the knowledge and skills to provide effective first aid can help reduce panic and create a sense of calm.

Learning and practicing first aid skills can also have a positive impact on mental health. Being prepared and knowing how to handle an emergency can reduce anxiety and stress levels, providing a sense of control and empowerment.

There are many ways to learn and practice first aid skills, including taking a course from a certified instructor, participating in online courses or tutorials, or practicing with a friend or family member. Regardless of the method, taking the time to learn and practice first aid skills can be a life-changing experience.

In conclusion, learning and practicing first aid skills is a vital skill set that can have a profound impact on an individual's life and the lives of those around them. Encouraging people to learn and practice first aid skills can empower them to take action in an emergency, create a sense of preparedness, and provide a valuable sense of control and empowerment.